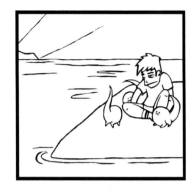

Down the F'n Tubes

an ode to fertility futility

Published by Tunnel Falls
www.facebook.com/downthefntubes

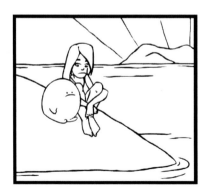

'Twas their third year of marriage, but this was a first.
Rick and Riley, let's be clear, were coitus well-versed...

They'd done missionary, doggy,
cow-girl reverse.
They'd spooned and they'd forked,
and they'd role-play rehearsed.

But tonight it was special.
Tonight they felt free.
'Cause tonight was their first night
without a goalie.

No condoms or spermicide.
No pills, diaphragms.
No hasty withdrawal,
catching spunk in his hands.

They had scheduled this night,
their first "timed-relation."
No sex just for sex—it was sex for creation!

"Think it took?" Riley asked,
as she pulled in her knees.
"There's no question," Rick said.
"Getting pregnant's a breeze.
All our friends and our siblings have had kids
with ease!"

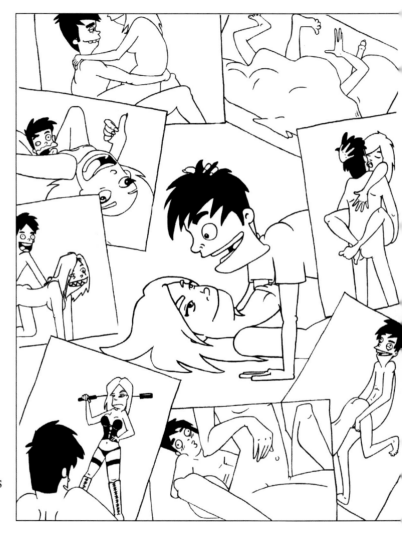

Rick and Riley went to sleep, their job now complete.
Any caveman can do it; it's no special feat.
Insert dick in vagina, and gametes will meet!

But as Rick slumbered off,
in an unconscious stream,
he felt something damp,
but 'twas not a wet dream.

He was getting a visit
from mythical beings:
The Almighty **Eets**,
The Protectors of Genes!

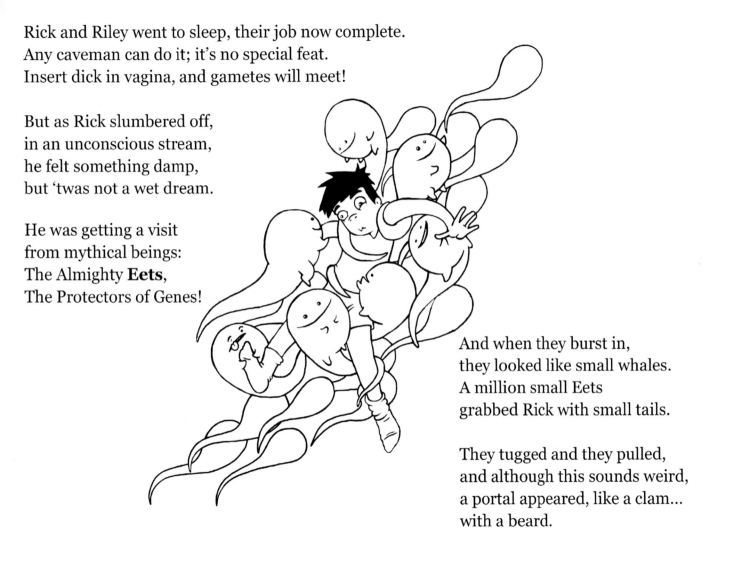

And when they burst in,
they looked like small whales.
A million small Eets
grabbed Rick with small tails.

They tugged and they pulled,
and although this sounds weird,
a portal appeared, like a clam...
with a beard.

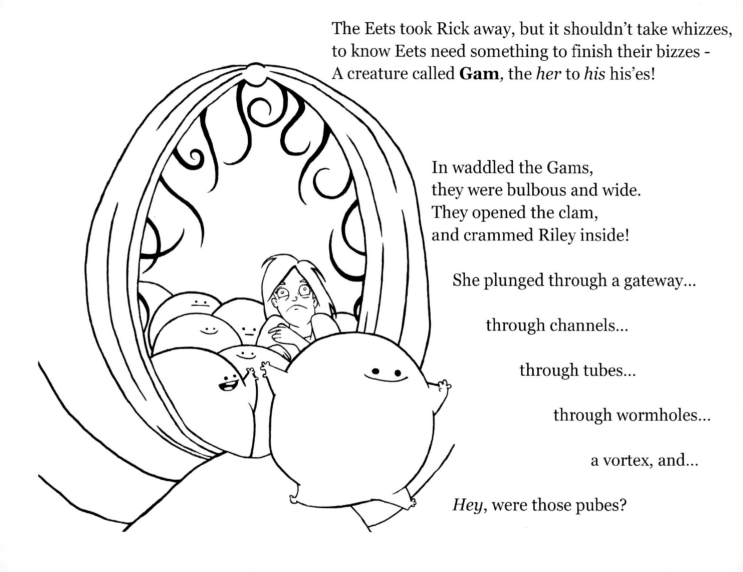

The Eets took Rick away, but it shouldn't take whizzes,
to know Eets need something to finish their bizzes -
A creature called **Gam**, the *her* to *his* his'es!

In waddled the Gams,
they were bulbous and wide.
They opened the clam,
and crammed Riley inside!

She plunged through a gateway...

through channels...

through tubes...

through wormholes...

a vortex, and...

Hey, were those pubes?

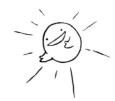

She was pushed on her tush, and gushed out on the sand,
surrounded by Gams, in a cold, barren land.

"Can you help us?" Gams pleaded.
"Oh, save us, oh please!
Our world grows so old,
and so cold that we'll freeze."

"Once a month, we send one,
floating into the sea.
There's an island out there,
that can grow baby trees.
It's teeming with life,
full of birds... and the bees!"

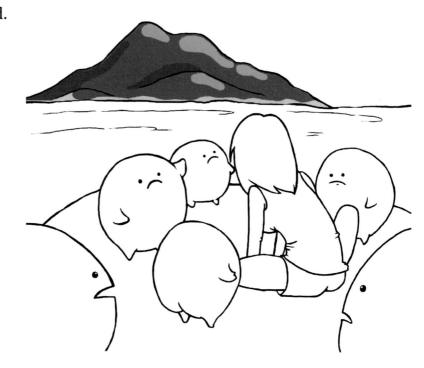

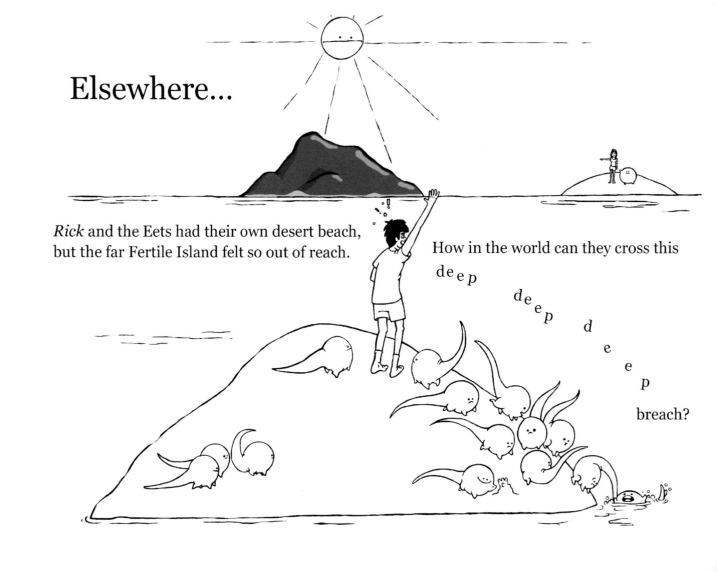

Elsewhere...

Rick and the Eets had their own desert beach,
but the far Fertile Island felt so out of reach.

How in the world can they cross this deep deep deep breach?

As Rick looked at the tides, "There's a time to this flow.
Just wait for my signal, then all of you go."

And so Rick watched his watch,
as they gathered 'round him.
When the cycle was right,
they were ordered to

"SWIM!"

A million burst forward,

then a million Eets more!

But Rick watched the island...

none had made it to shore.

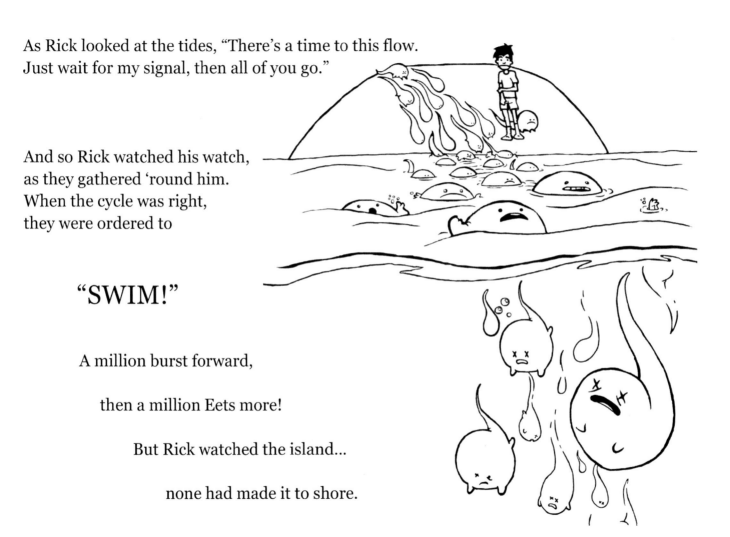

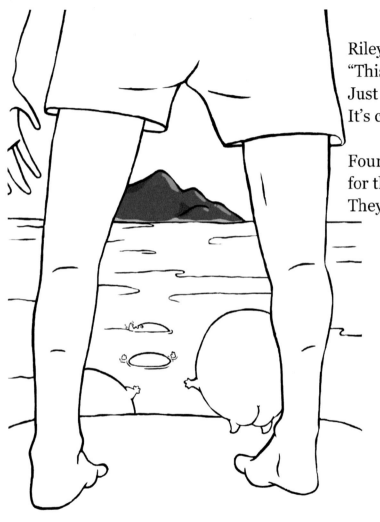

Riley stared at the sea and said,
"This isn't tough.
Just send in more Gams.
It's clear *one's* not enough."

Four Gams were picked,
for their strength and bulbosity.
They dove in and swam with unmatched ferocity.

But when the Gams approached land,
they were slammed by a flood.
These waves *weren't* of water.
No, this flood was of BLOOD!

"What is this?!" Riley asked.

All the rest bowed their heads.
"Every month this land sheds,
and the water turns red."

And Riley then knew that the four Gams were dead.

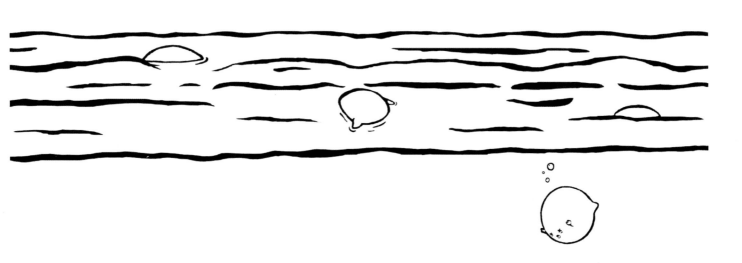

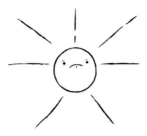

As the blood sloshed about, it was messy as fuck.
It took days to flow out. This period did suck.

So they waited...

... and waited...

... for waters to clear.

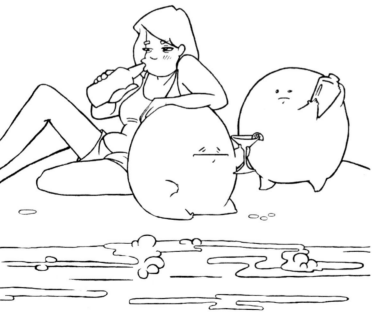

This annoying occurrence
came often that year.

But during those times,
she could at least have a beer.

When new water flowed in, and the island regrew,
they were done jerking off, they knew just what to do:

They both picked their teams—on strength and agility,
on shape, on their size, and on their motility.

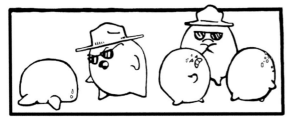

Then they trained them and drugged them
until they were strong,
strong enough to survive in the sea for so long.

And when the timing was right, they tried to
swim fast...

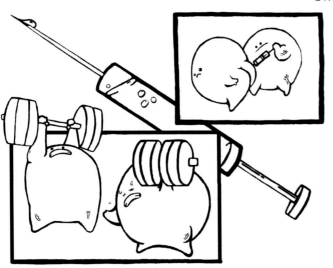

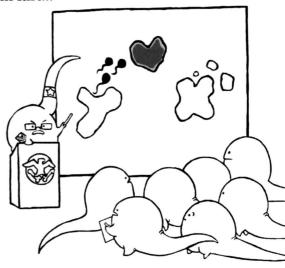

But for reasons unknown, they just did not last.

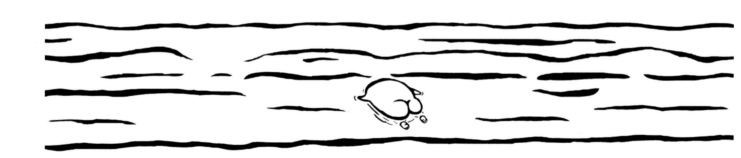

No one wanted to quit, and so another month passed.

"Here's the plan," Rick said, "We'll reach that island, but FAST."

"We will build us a boat, packed with all it can hold,
we will cross this here moat, and release the payload!"

So they banged and they nailed,
this brand new erection.

They boarded and sailed—
it was a Sea Men collection!

But the sea was too wide. Yet again they all died.
Neither side could survive the strength of these tides.

The Gams were all tired, the Eets all annoyed,
as month after month, all their friends were destroyed.

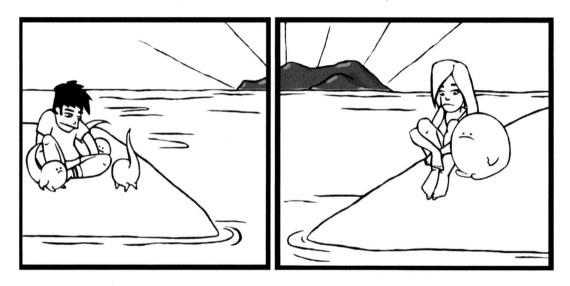

Soon the months became years, and then some years more.
As the time ticked away, their psyches grew sore.

With each passing year, there was less chance to win.
The island grew smaller; their numbers grew thin.

Other islands and seas won with ease at this game.
As their own failure mounted, a new feeling came...

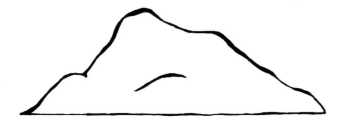

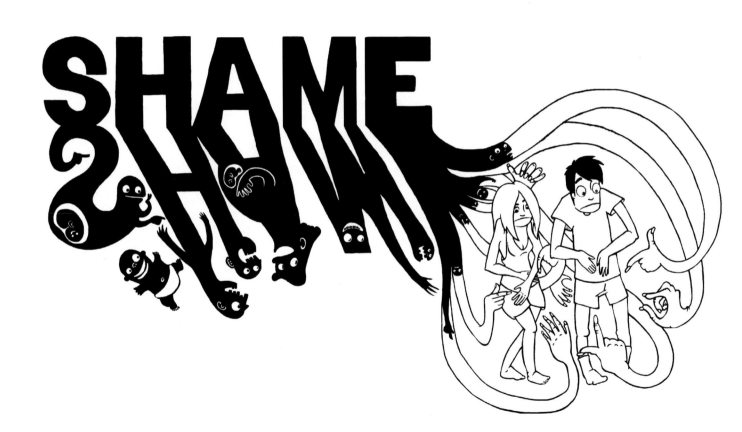

Was **SHE** to blame?

Was **HE** to blame?

Maybe his *old* dame wouldn't be so lame.

Maybe her *old* flame wouldn't have poor aim.

FUCK
SHAME

If their success will depend on just her and him,
then fuck all this waiting—they were going to swim!

With a Gam in her hands and the Eets on his head,
through the sea they'd carry them *themselves* there instead.

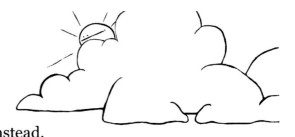

But the ocean fought back. It was hard to resist.
They dodged polyps, 'metriosis, and a few cysts!

The waves swelled to high heights, and boy was it scary.
But they held on tight—they couldn't bear to miscarry.

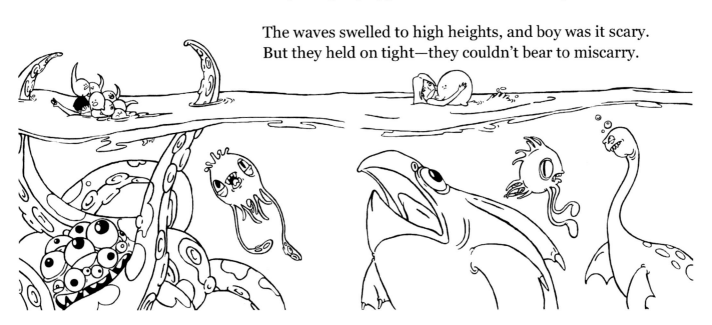

And just when success felt less than believable...
When reaching the shore still seemed unachievable...
They gave one final push and the inconceived ...

WAS CONCEIVABLE!

Then Gam ran to Eet,
it was love at first sight!
They wrapped up each other,
and held on so tight.

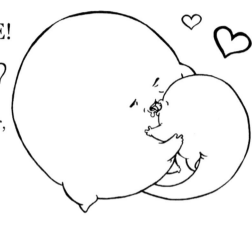

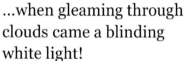

...when gleaming through
clouds came a blinding
white light!

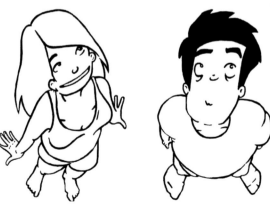

When the light dissipated, they had a surprise,
'cause instead of their friends, stood a tree there (pint-sized).

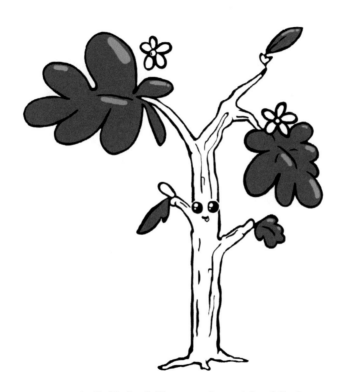

A delightfully, perfect, ideal baby tree.
The exact kind of tree that a new tree should be.

Rick and Riley then knew life would not be the same.
They decorated the land and picked out some names.

They watered the roots, gave it plenty of light.
They read to it, loved it, talked to it at night.

But by chance one day, baby tree just stopped growing.
And they saw, in the breeze, a red leaf was blowing...

They tried not to worry 'bout the red leaf they found,

but an hour went by...

...and there were more on the ground.

There was no way to save it and nothing to do.
They just had to brave it 'til the process was through.

It's hard to conceive after so many tries,
that they must now grieve this unwelcome surprise.

So they sat on the beach, and looked out with dismay,
as their long-fought-for tree quickly withered away.

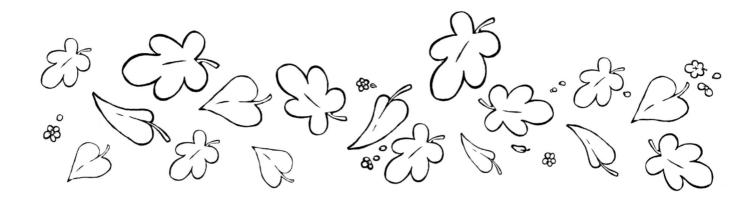

They were damaged and broken. At life they had failed.
While all other lands, without trying, prevailed.

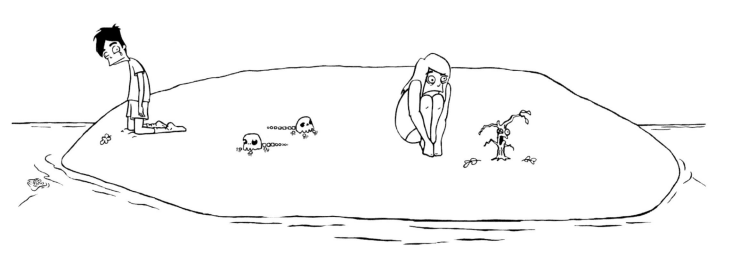

On the island they sat, feeling shame and defeat,
and asked, "Why the fuck can't our Gams and Eets meet???"

Rick and Riley both sighed and then they said, "Screw it.
If others make trees, we may as well view it."

They walked up the hill, gazing far as can be.
They saw other lands, other seas, other trees.

Other Gams, other Eets crossed *their* seas like a breeze.

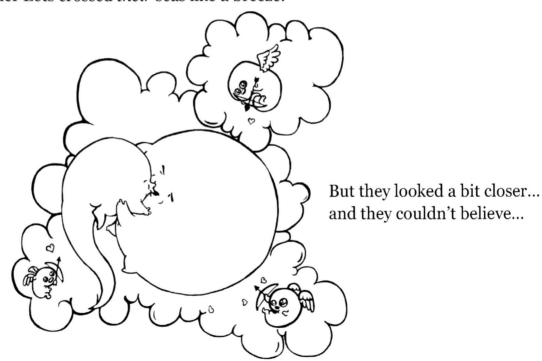

But they looked a bit closer...
and they couldn't believe...

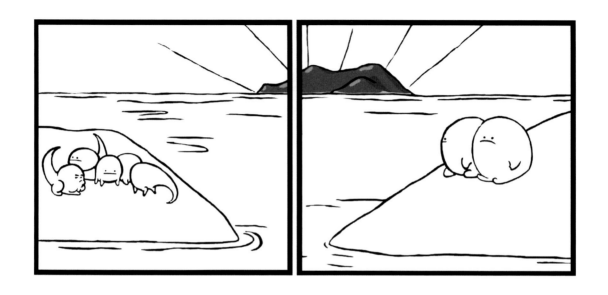

Other Gams were all tired. *Other* Eets were annoyed.
Other Gams' and Eets' efforts sank into the void.

Yet...

Some people had trees but their islands weren't green.
They sprouted their seeds with unconventional means:

At last some succeeded to get their tree seeded.
They didn't stop swimming; perseverance was needed!

Some found strangers' trees—raising them was an option.
This old strategy was sure ripe for adoption!

And still others found comfort tree-sitting for friends.
(While maintaining the freedom to sleep on weekends.)

Yet for millions out there, trees cannot be achieved,
through no fault of theirs. Yes, it's hard to conceive.

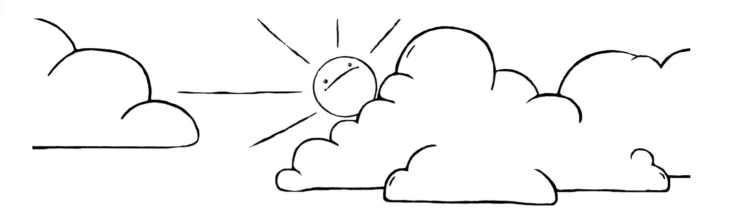

And Riley and Rick?

Well, they haven't stopped swimming.
A great life together was still just beginning.

They may have a tree, but then again maybe not.
But they'll never forget or regret what they've got.

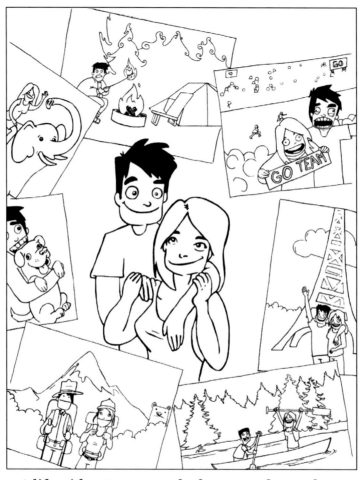

A life without trees can be happy and complete.
Because sometimes it's hard to get gametes to meet.

Made in the USA
Monee, IL
22 February 2020

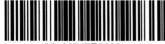